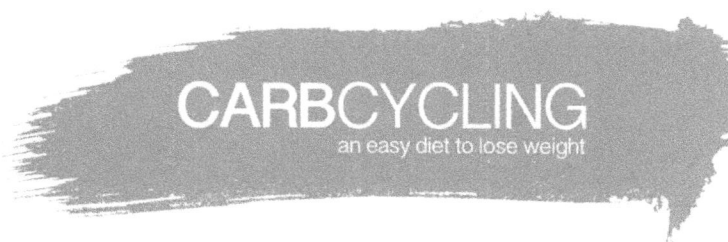

CARBCYCLING
an easy diet to lose weight

Frank Tolbert

©2019 Blanco Publishing

ISBN-13: 978-1-09922-153-8

INTRODUCTION

Carbohydrate Cycling Diet, or for shorter, Carb Cycling Diet is a type of diet where amounts of carbs and calories by and large differed from day to day.

Carb Cycling Diet is by and large fundamentally the same as Weight Loss Liquid Diet as far as calories, macronutrient substance and number of meals – Weight Loss Liquid Diet utilizes fluid meals with week after week/every day cheat supper being healthy strong feast, while Carb Cycling Diet uses typical healthy substantial meals in light of substance and segment control.

Only realizing what food to eat, those that would ensure your body gets the supplements it needs, isn't enough to accomplish a fit and healthy body. Diet would never be without exercise; they are a pair alluded to as fitness sustenance, the blend of both. Those that exercise progressively, like athletes, require more food and supplements so their body could stay aware of all the physical exercises they experience.

Carbohydrates, albeit erroneously kept away from by individuals on diets, are useful particularly if you embrace physical exercises or sports like a dashing, ball of playing badminton. This is because these "carbs" produce the blood sugar in the body, this blood sugar, which is all the more regularly referred to as glucose, is put away as glycogen in the muscles. Glycogen gives the energy a person needs to perform such exercises. Without glucose, a person can undoubtedly feel depleted and exhausted. Some diet junkies think that they "sweat off the fat" in their body, yet as a rule, they sweat off the glycogen first and after that the fat.

While carbohydrates are significant for brisk exercises, fats are required by the body while doing long continuance exercises like cycling or running long distance races. A healthy person does not have zero fat in their authority; they have fat and in certainty, use them as a wellspring of energy amid their exercises. Without fat, your body tends to utilize the energy put away in the proteins. This isn't ideal since the body needs these proteins to repair the muscles.

Nutrients and minerals, although not energy producers are significant for other wellbeing capacities. They give the calcium that reinforces the bones, the iron that helps in transporting oxygen all through the body, and a few minerals like potassium help in the guideline of water in the body amid thorough workouts.

Information in regard to fitness nourishment is essential to figure out what specific food to eat or drink before you manage your exercise schedule. Around 3-6 hours before you exercise, it is advisable that you consume a full, healthy supper. A couple of hours before actually working cut, you ought to consume food that is rich in carbohydrates, or even better complex carbohydrates. This food type can give a large amount of carbohydrate which can accommodate more energy amid your exercises. Never neglect to drink water, amid and after your exercise. Sweating makes the water in the body dissipate. An individual must supplant this lost fluid immediately to avert dehydration.

Remember that excessively little or a lot of exercises can be awful. Be specific with your exercise regime; ensure it fits the type of way of life you lead. If you are already worn out from work throughout the day, try exercises which are not all that intense like short runs. Continuously eat a balanced diet; after all, it is the other portion of fitness nourishment. Never under any circumstance, skip meals to ensure that your body is all around sustained and drink bunches of water and fluid. This ensures the body stays fit as a fiddle regardless of whether you are working out.

CHAPTER ONE

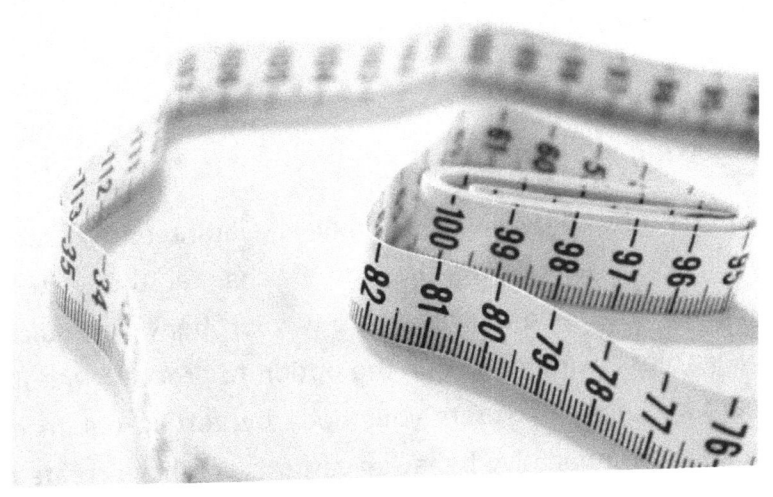

What Is Carb Cycling

Carb Cycling is actually as it sounds cycling your carbs. You may recollect the "low-carb" diet that was a prevailing national fashion quite a while prior. People got results, for some time in any event. The main problem with low-carb diets is that they are meant as temporary diets you can't eat that way until the end of time. Your body can't eat that way, as it needs carbs for everyday work. Indeed, in all honesty, your body requires carbs.

At that point, there's the opposite end of the range, the individuals who advocate high-carb diets. While high-carb diets help to speed your metabolism, they are not ideal for weight-loss, as there is certainly not an adequate deficiency to enable you to shed the pounds. This is the place carb-cycling comes in.

Resetting your body

While various prevailing fashion diets guarantee to "reset" your body, everything they do is channel the water, supplements, and nutrients from your body for quick weight loss, without having the option to proceed with it. Carb cycling truly resets your body by getting out from under those negative behavior patterns you have created, while in the meantime showing your body new, better propensities. It's a simple, one-step process and an excellent plan for a lifetime of wellbeing. Carb cycling is easy, inexpensive, and you can do everything all alone. There is no compelling reason to spend lots of money on a program or exceptional nourishment. There are resources you can buy to help you on your adventure. However, you can prevail without these also.

How it functions

The "enchantment" of carb cycling is that is works by giving your body both the fuel it needs to build metabolism and making calorie shortfalls to expand fat loss. Days are turned between high-carb days and low-carb days. Did you realize your body is intended to eat multiple meals a day? Three meals were not a regular event until the mechanical age. Or maybe, to maximize weight loss and keep your metabolism consuming, the best schedule is one that eats five times each day, or at regular intervals. This may seem like a lot; however, following a couple of days of eating along these lines, your body will wind up hungry and need to eat like clockwork. Eating three meals a day will be a struggle, as it is a lot of nourishment, particularly promptly in the day, be that as it may, it will work. This joined with pre-portioned meals and a regular exercise routine, including cardio and weight preparing, will consume fat and tone muscle!

The Truth About Diet Myths

How would we know what we know? Often, our knowledge originates from repetition and stories. In childhood, we call them fairy tales or sleep time stories. They interest or engage and have with the occasional good exercise. However, as grown-ups, these stories or myths can be harmful when we begin settling on decisions dependent on their often mistaken information.

This often occurs in food choices, particularly with regards to shedding pounds. Through repetition, even incorrect information can penetrate our thoughts and impede weight misfortune objectives. The issue is, numerous ideas or stories surround weight misfortune get rehashed so often, they become believable.

We should look at the science behind a portion of these old stories:

Myth #1: Initial weight misfortune on diet plans originates from lost water weight.

There is no water stockpiling organ in the human body that exhausts after dieting. The proponents of this fallacy usually argue that the breakdown of glycogen in the liver, a regular event in the body of a dieter, causes the arrival of water. The human liver weighs around 3 pounds, and glycogen represents just about 10% of this. Along these lines, water from the liver could only add to not exactly a large portion of a pound misfortune, and that is if the majority of its weight were water.

The fallacy mongers further recommend that the breakdown results of fat metabolism discharge water. However, for the technically disapproved, the vast majority of these chemical reactions use water initially, as opposed to discharge it.

Myth #2: Skipping meals is a practical way to get thinner.

When you skirt a meal, your body utilizes put away sugar atoms which have been changed over to glycogen. These stores are in the liver and muscle tissue. Once these are gone, your body turns to other nutrient sources for its constant vitality needs. After avoiding a meal under this circumstance, your body shifts into a "fasting" metabolism, which leads to protein breakdown.

If you are eating as per evolutionary rules, that is, the correct combination of foods for your body's plan, you would break down fat, instead of protein, by NOT skipping lunch.

Myth #3: The Food Pyramid is a decent way to eat to keep up a healthy weight.

The U.S. Department of Agriculture discharged the Food Pyramid in 1980 and released a refreshed form in mid-

2005. The Pyramid advocates a diet with plenty of bread, grains, rice, pasta, vegetables, and natural products. However, decisions about food choices are much more complicated than following a list of suggested foods. Our food choices are the result of a combination of body signals, cultural influences, propensities, occasions, people, feelings, and convictions. Since the introduction of The Food Pyramid, obesity has become of pandemic proportion. It appears to be economically driven agricultural promotion isn't serving public health.

Myth #4: Eating a low-fat diet is the best way to get in shape.

Low-fat diets have been supported throughout the previous 20 years, and the fat substance of the American diet has diminished marginally amid this time. However, the obesity rate has dramatically increased. Why? Part of the reason is that a low-fat diet isn't the right fuel mix for the way the human body was planned. More than millions of years of evolution, our metabolic pathways created. The original diet comprised for the most of available vegetation, seasonally constrained leafy foods, and foods wealthy in protein and fat.

Myth #5: Counting calories is fundamental to healthy eating and weight misfortune.

The human body needs around 11-12 calories for each pound of weight per day to keep up its present importance. For a 200-pound person, this would be approximately 2400 calories. About 3500 calories are eaten for every pound of body weight. In this way, to shed 10 pounds, a dieter would need to ingest 35,000 fewer calories. It would follow, that by eating 500 fewer calories a day, it would assume control more than two months to shed those 10 pounds. However, for the vast majority, this noteworthy calorie limitation is awkward and unsustainable. For anyone who has attempted a reduced calorie diet, they are familiar with how difficult along these lines of life can be. What do you do when at 5 PM all the day's calories are gone, and you are yet eager?

The body unexpectedly processes various nutrients. It isn't the total amount of food eaten that leads to weight misfortune or increase. It is the proportion of different nutrients and the shift to fat consuming metabolism that is significant.

Sadly, contending interests depend on these "certainties" and help sustain their reality. To shed pounds, you should advise yourself regarding how your body developed and your body's process of metabolism if you need to know how you ought to eat and how to get in shape. Trusting diet myths will keep you in the cycle of the sequential dieter.

THE TRUTH ABOUT CARB CYCLING

It should not shock the rest of the country that the number one thing at the forefront of everyone's thoughts is how to shed that 20, 30, or even 50 pounds. Theory, after theory, after method, after theory attempt to help turn around the onset of weight gain; however, never truly hit the imprint. Regardless of whether it is because the theory is defective, or it is part of the business model, nobody can make sure.

One such theory is the possibility of 'carb cycling.'

This is nothing new and has been around for a long while. Professional bodybuilders like to utilize carb cycling to increase mass throughout their preparation. For most it does some amazing things, however, for some it opens itself up to a host of different issues.

Carb cycling is a practice that includes severely cutting the measure of carbohydrates expend for a timeframe somewhere in the range of three to seven days pursued by multi-day or two of expanded carbohydrate consumption.

Although this method of eating has been around some time, it is as yet a defective framework.

When we eat carbohydrates, the sugar or glucose makes it into our bloodstream where some of it is retained into our muscle and fat tissues, and some are scorched off all the while.

Presently if our admission of carbohydrates is expanded, at that point we are left with excess sugar in our blood, and when that happens, our body's reaction is to discharge insulin to help flush that sugar once more into different places on our body.

Am I not catching this' meaning for you?

All things considered, if you are proceeding to exhaust your carb admission and, at that point significantly increment it then the insulin in your body will be streaming always and if you do it more than once over an extensive stretch of time, at that point you risk your body constructing a protection from it.

One thing that these bodybuilders overlook is that insulin is a 'fat-putting away' hormone. It takes that extra glycogen and powers it into your muscles, and when those fill up, it begins putting away it in the most noticeably terrible spots possible on your body as fat. This is the reason you will some professional bodybuilders or guys preparing for active man competitions that have a tad of a gut on them. This is their body putting away those extra sugars that they have devoured.

Anyway, the bottom line is carb cycling entirely hazardous regardless of anything else. If you keep yo-yo-ing your blood sugar here and there, at that point your body will need to keep on controlling it. The best method of practice is to keep it as even as could reasonably be expected. This will forestall excess fat storage just like those nasty cravings when your blood sugar crashes because of insulin carrying out its responsibility.

Carb Cycling - Is it Necessary?
What is carb cycling or re-nourishing?

When you are endeavoring to get in shape, its regularly a good idea to control your carb intake. Not because carbs are bad, but since carbs (like pasta and rice) are delicious and effectively accessible. We regularly will, in general, gorge them and pack on the calories. By and by, I have had outstanding accomplishment by controlling my carb intake for dinners. You are bound to indulge carbs amid dinner than some other feast. Supplanting a regular high carb dinner with a salad will spare you hundreds of calories daily!!!

However, if your lower caloric intake proceeds for quite a while, your body will adjust to it by lowering your metabolism. For example, If your body required 2500 daily calories to keep up weight and you just ate 2000 calories, your body would at first lose a pound every week. Do this sufficiently long, and your body will lower your daily maintenance level to coordinate 2000 calories.

What happens at that point? You quit losing weight!

So the rationale goes you ought to change your calorie utilization to shield the body from adjusting to a lower calorie diet. How would you do it? You cycle your carb/calorie intake to increment or diminishing the number of calories you devour. A few people cycle daily, others cycle every 3-4 days.

There are many variations of carb cycling or calorie cycling. For example, you have a salad for dinner 3 days straight. At that point on the fourth day, you have a serving of pasta or rice with your dinner. Or on the other hand, you may add some dessert to your dinner. This will raise the calorie intake by 400-500 calories for that day, and afterward, you rehash the cycle. This "crest" in calories keeps the body from hindering the metabolism.

Would it be a good idea for you to utilize carb cycling to get in shape?

Well, the appropriate response isn't as necessary. Everything depends on how much weight you need to lose and how strongly you have been working out.

Overlook carb cycling if you...

...have more than 20 pounds to lose, you can concentrate on making calorie deficiency on a weekly premise through sustenance and exercise.

...are effectively getting thinner every week with your current eating regimen and exercise plan. Try not to fix what isn't broken.

You should utilize carb cycling if you...

...have less than 20 pounds to lose. The leaner and fitter you are, the more your body will oppose shedding pounds. So you should trick your body into shedding those last couple of pounds.

...Have quit shedding pounds. if you are already eating smaller portions; at that point, cutting calories further can reverse discharge. You could take a stab at practicing more, however sooner or later that won't be enough.

If you are keen on a program that takes out all the mystery for you, I profoundly prescribe Tom Venuto's BFFM. I have been following this program for over a year, and I have effectively dropped more than 12-13% body fat and more than 35 pounds.

For the individuals who have quit shedding pounds, increment your calorie intake for a week. One week of higher calories will give your body a chance to adjust to a higher metabolic rate. At that point drop your calorie intake back to what it was, really going after a couple of weeks and rehash. Another trick is to exchange lower calorie days with higher calorie days. Ensure your higher calorie days are not an excuse to overeat, however, eat with some restraint!

Does Carb Cycling Work? Carb cycling has become a significant buzzword in the weight loss industry. Otherwise called Carb Rotating, this has become a method which many people are utilizing to get their weight loss process going quickly and continuously.

What is carb cycling, and does it truly work?

Carb cycling is an eating method wherein you modify the measure of carb calories that you expend starting with one day then onto the next. You slip in low carb days sometimes yet when they come standard carb days. What this accomplishes is 2 things: First, the little carb days help you to make a calorie shortage expected to get in shape. Second, the cycling or carb pivoting causes you to shield your digestion from backing off as it regularly does when we lessen our general calorie consumption. The metabolic impact encourages us to keep shedding pounds far into the future.

Does carb cycling work? Like some other method, it is anything but a 100% secure arrangement. Likewise, it is easy to misunderstand in by not eating at optimal hours or notwithstanding eating the wrong sort of carbs. Be that as it may, done right, it tends to be exceptionally successful. People are detailing losing as much as 15 pounds per month with it. It is additionally an eating method which is recommended by different nutritionists. An additional benefit is that this weight loss method doesn't require you to starve yourself senseless as it's generally easy to stick to for a long span and to keep up the weight loss once you accomplish it.

Make a point to pursue a specialist laid carb cycling plan, so you don't finish up treating it terribly.

CHAPTER TWO

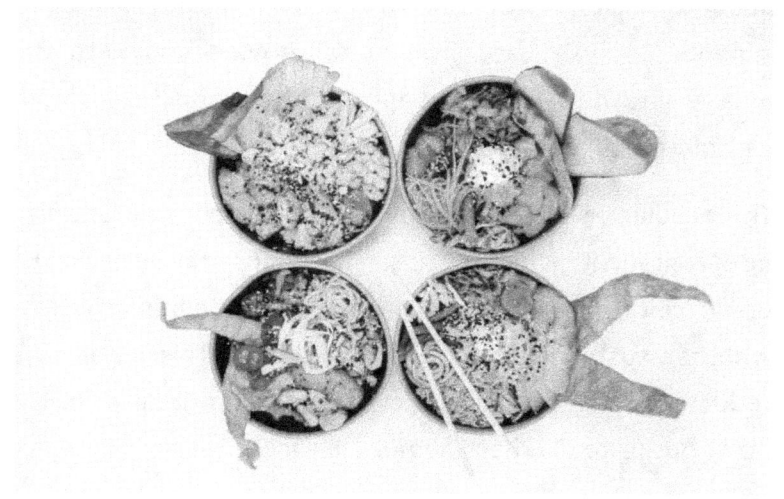

How Does Carb Cycling Really Work?

Carb Cycling is the basis of many weight misfortune methods and used in various forms by individuals who wish to lose fat, form muscles, get conditioned, and for many more wellness objectives. In any case, how does carb cycling work and for what reason is it such a popular method?

Carbs make up most of the calories we eat. Carbs are found in anything from sugar, through bread and pasta, to foods grown from the ground. There is no shortage of carbs around us. The problem is the way to eat carbs to burn body fat faster appropriately.

This is the place carb cycling comes in. Essentially, you need to ensure that your body utilizes the carbs you expend. By best use, I mean to provide you with the energy you have to work appropriately and to workout without putting on weight or body fat.

The problem is that our body gives close consideration to how we feed it. When we endeavor to lose fat by chopping down calories or carbs, it immediately begins to stress whether sustenance is over to get rare. This leads to a reduction in digestion, and a slower fat burning rate, the polar opposite of what you need to occur.

This is the place carb cycling comes in. Carb cycling (otherwise called carb rotation) is finished by exchanging up the number of carbs that you eat starting with one day then onto the next. What you're essentially attempting to do is to "trap" your body, so it never knows precisely how you're going to bolster it.

For example, you may cause your body to bring its digestion up in the desire for a lot of carbs; however, then you feed it a bit. This causes your body to burn a lot of calories, although you're just putting in a little amount. This is only one of the tricks required, as there are many. The key is to have low, medium, and high carb days to keep your body "speculating" and your fat burning rate as high as could be allowed.

Carb cycling is popular because it produces results, and it is an easy and possible fat misfortune method. To be sure, it can even be used to develop more significant muscle mass as it is a system that can be tweaked for many wellness objectives.

If you wind up attempting diet designs again and again and neglecting to shed pounds regularly, you ought to consider cycling your carbs. It might be precisely what you need.

CARB CYCLING FOR WOMEN

Have you achieved a plateau in your eating regimen regime where the loss of weight appears to have ceased? If you have, at that point isn't it about time like such a significant number of other women around the world you attempted the eating routine known as carb cycling. With regards to carb cycling for women, it can assist you with losing those additional pounds all the more viable without really requiring you to wipe out sustenance that are basic to how your body consumes truth.

So precisely what is carb cycling? With this specific eating routine, you are required for a time of 2 to 3 days decrease the number of carbs that you consume. At that point for the next 2 to 3 days, you increment the number of carbs you consume once more.

What this eating regimen does is helps on the lower carb days you utilize the fat put away in the body to give it vitality as you work out; thus, fat gets signed off more rapidly. While on the different days when you consume more carbs, this is going to help replenish the vitality you have lost while ensuring that when you are not doing any sort of physical movement your digestion still capacities at ideal levels.

If you do utilize this eating regimen to help get more fit dissimilar to others, there are no exacting rules for you to stick to. With this one, it is observing how your body reacts when you roll out the improvements in the levels of carbs you eat will decide how successful it is. You may find that you are someone who can eat carbs containing more starch as opposed to the stringy ones to accomplish your weight reduction objectives.

How to Develop a Carb Cycling Diet

Carb cycling is an incredible weight reduction device. Before figuring out how to practice carb cycling, it's vital to build up the blueprint for a healthy diet.

A healthy diet is a sensible diet. Eat in any event 3 square meals a day. Be mindful of including carbohydrate, protein, and fat source with every meal.

A meal can run anyplace from a plunk down supper to a little tidbit like a banana. The word that I like to utilize while portraying portion measure is sensible. Is it accurate to say that you are eating until you are full? If so, you are overeating. Do you feel hungry in the wake of eating? Bump up the calories.

Notice that I don't utilize the "D" word. Diet has a negative meaning. It says "limitation," and whenever that we feel confined, we will engage in general revolutionary. Disregard that word and focus on what you need: a leaner, healthier body.

To streamline our performance, it's essential to fuel up with the best possible sustenance.

Some phenomenal dull carbohydrate sources are oatmeal, sweet potatoes, potatoes, dark-colored rice, wild rice, entire wheat pasta, whole wheat bread, cream of wheat, Kashi oat, entire wheat saltines, and destroyed wheat oat. Fruits are likewise incorporated into this category.

Lean protein sources are chicken, turkey, beans, skim milk, whey protein blend, casein protein blend, fish, egg whites, and soy protein.

Solid fats are typical nutty spread, olive oil, flax seed oil, safflower oil, almonds, and walnuts.

Green carbohydrates are your green veggies.

Pursue this carb cycling program.

Day #1 - Eat a dull carbohydrate source with every meal up until 6:00 PM or thereabouts. After 6:00 PM, meals should consist of a protein and fat source.

Day #2 - Eat a dull carbohydrate source with every meal up until 6:00 PM or something like that. After 6:00 PM, meals should consist of a protein and fat source.

Day #3 - Eat a green carbohydrate source within any event 3 meals. Bump up the protein and fat utilization a smidgen today. Eat an extra meal.

Day #4 - Repeat Day #1

Day #5 - Repeat Day #2

Day #6 - Repeat Day #3

Repeat this carb cycling pattern of 2 higher carb days/1 lower carb day for a couple of weeks. Toss in 2 consecutive quieter carb days following 2 weeks. Change the diet to make it intriguing and to keep your body speculating. The human body is tremendously efficient, and you have to deceive it to keep your program viable.

Be sensible! Be restrained with your carb cycling routine however realize that you are qualified for desserts or whatever you want most. If you are occupied with an exercise program, you can stand to eat junk sustenance a couple of times a week. Try not to beat yourself up over a carb-up one to two times every week.

I'm convinced that the feelings which we partner with nourishment are the factor which decides whether they influence our body unfavorably. I used to show and needed to keep razor-lean physical make-up. I tallied each calorie. I named certain nourishments tremendous and unfortunate. I would feel horrible if I genuinely overate. I wanted to work out for 3 hours to consume off the meal.

Intelligence has empowered me to see the craziness in this kind of reasoning. Presently I wouldn't fret when I eat those 4 packages of Little Debbies. I've discovered that if I remain sensible more often than not, my weight will keep on dropping. I don't feel bad about eating junk sustenance any longer. I appreciate it! If you don't feel bad about eating junk sustenance, it won't influence you. Trust me on this one!

Play around with this carb cycling program. Try not to approach it with the last chance attitude. Be grateful for the changes that you find in your body, and you'll be bound to carry on with a sound way of life. You'll look great and feel incredible.

Getting Started With a Low Carb Diet Plan

Once you're at long last settled on the decision to get thinner, and you've chosen you to need to attempt a low carb diet plan, the critical step is finished. All you have to do now is necessarily begin. How about taking a gander at what your first several days of a low carb diet plan may resemble?

One Day of your low carb diet plan should begin with some firm decisions. First you choose you will get in the shape of course, and second, you decide to go with a low carb diet plan to achieve that weight misfortune. Next, however, you are to pick which low carb diet plan you mean to follow. Three popular ones incorporate the Atkins low carb diet plan, The South Beach low carb diet plan, and The Glycemic Index low carb diet plan.

Notwithstanding which plan you pick, the objective is to lower your everyday admission of carbs and begin truly losing a portion of the additional weight and fat your body has been clutching. On day one, choose which low carb diet plan, you will follow and acclimate yourself with how that low carb diet plan functions explicitly.

second Day of your low carb diet plan will include planning and arrangement. First, you have to get out your cupboards, washroom, fridge, and cooler. Hurl out or give away any high carb, high sugar content foods that you won't eat with your low carb diet plan.

Most low carb diet plans don't allow you to have certain foods in the first week or two on the program, yet you can bite by bit include those foods in later. You may end up disposing of foods you have right now that aren't overly high in carbs, however, aren't yet allowed for the beginning of your low carb diet plan. Try not to give up. However, many of these foods will be included back in throughout the next couple of weeks.

Next, you will need to make a list of what you will eat for in any event the next week. Incorporate dinners, snacks, and fluids; at that point, make a shopping list for those things. Last, however not least, you will go to the store and purchase the majority of the foods on your list.

Making these strides will enable you to begin directly with the low carb diet plan based on your personal preference, and it allows you to adhere to the best possible rules and guidelines for that plan also.

Day three of your low carb diet plan is the point at which you will change how you eat. You don't need to hold up until this day, to begin with, your new low carb diet plan. However, it very well may be useful to begin new toward the beginning of a modern day, rather than beginning amidst a day. Starting your new low carb diet plan toward the beginning of a brand-new day will make you feel progressively dedicated to the idea as opposed to feeling like it was a hasty decision on the off the cuff.

Day three is a decent day to complete a touch of cooking as well. By getting ready foods that are allowed amid this beginning stage of your low carb diet plan, you're ensuring you will dependably have something great to eat that is anything but difficult to snatch and go. One of the biggest pitfalls of most low carb diet plans is that you have to cook the right foods for your specific scenario. Furthermore, if you don't have something cooked and prepared when you need it, you're bound to tumble off the project and harm your weight misfortune endeavors.

The next several days of your low carb diet plan probably won't be the best. You will experience sugar and starch cravings, you might be worn out and torpid, and you may have cerebral pains or mellow dazedness. These are on the whole standard symptoms of beginning a low carb diet plan because your body is wiping out all the additional starches, sugars, and garbage that has been stored up for a spell. Your body is experiencing withdrawal from the lack of sugar that it's utilized to, and these early days on your low carb diet plan are while having pre-cooked foods is most significant, because you're at a higher danger of stopping when you're not feeling admirable.

Once those couple of days of the withdrawal are finished. However, you will in all respects likely be excited with the aftereffects of picking a low carb diet plan. You'll have more energy, you won't feel as bloated, and you may even notice garments are now begun to fit all the more freely as well!

CHAPTER THREE

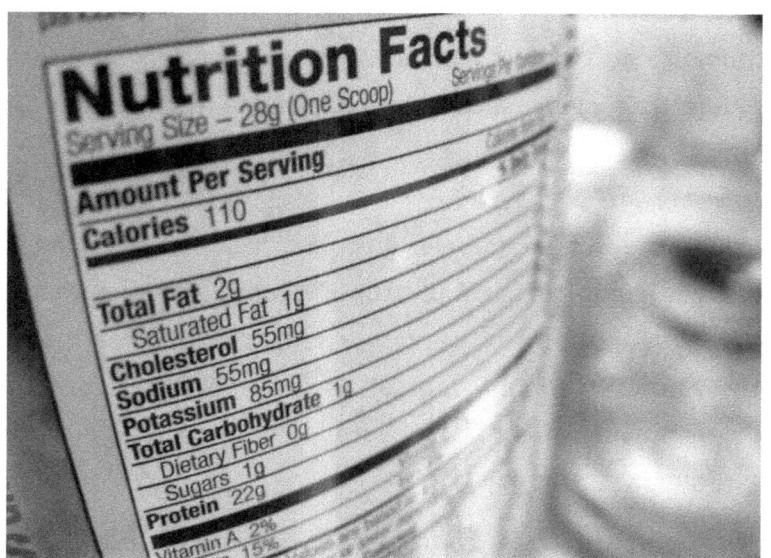

Carb Cycling Diet Tip

Low-calorie diets are a great way to peel off fat from your waist. However, it isn't sufficient. In this book, I need to go over how carb cycling can get you that ripped a set of 6 pack abs that you need so awful.

Generally, a low-calorie diet will come to the heart of the matter where you can see the best 4 abs on your midriff. You can get your body fat % down drastically by tallying calories and utilizing low-calorie diets, yet to cross the end goal you have to accomplish more.

The most common way to approach carb cycling is to have your most massive carb days on the days when you are training the hardest and lower carb days on your less severe training days. On your heavy training days, you are going to need to center the majority of your calories for right around your training period since this is the point at which your body needs them the most. On these big days, you are going to need to stun the body to animate the digestion and furnish you with vitality. On lower carb days you will be restricting yourself to generally eating protein dinners, with minimal measures of dietary fats just as carbohydrates.

When you are at last serious about getting a set of ripped abs, at that point the #1 activity is investigated your eating routine. If you are not eating the right way, it will be near impossible to see those lower abs. Use carb cycling to enable you to accomplish your 6 pack objectives. To get that highly characterized level of conditioning, you should venture up your eating regimen program and truly drive yourself to get the most extreme outcomes. If you time your carb cycling the right way, you can get yourself ripped in no time, at whatever point you need.

How to Do Carb Cycling

Carb cycling refers to an eating regimen that depends on cycling between days of high carbohydrate admission and days of low carbohydrate consumption. This concept was created in the bodybuilding industry, yet many games professionals likewise discovered that this technique can be exceptionally viable for healthy weight misfortune when combined with a proper exercise schedule.

Figuring out How to Carb Cycle

1 Pick a technique. There is no one right way to carb cycle. People utilize different carb cycling plans to meet their various needs and objectives. In this manner, you ought to pick a carb cycling plan that suits you.

- If you need to get more fit, for example, you should need to complete a plan that includes low-carb days for five days every week and afterward, have two high-carb days.
- Then again, if you are hoping to pick up muscle, you should need to attempt an all the more even blend of four high carb days and three low carb days.
- As an example, the "work of art" carb cycling schedule includes exchanging for 6 days every week between high-and low-carbs. On the seventh day, you get the chance to have a "cheat" day

where you don't have to screen your calorie and carb consumption so carefully.

2 **Decide your carb and calorie objectives.** As a general standard, on this diet, women should plan to take in around 1,200 calories every day, and men should prepare for about 1,500 calories on low-carb days. On high carb days, you'll eat slightly more calories.

- Another general standard to remember when beginning is that on high-carb days you should intend to consume about 1.5 grams of carbs per pound of body weight. So, if you weigh 150 pounds, you would need to consume 225 grams of carbohydrates. On low-carb days, you should attempt to dodge carbohydrate-rich foods, and stick to foods that are high in protein.

3 **Space out your days equally.** It's important to attempt to keep a balanced schedule, which includes spreading out your high-end low-carb days with the goal that you don't have such a large number of that day consecutive. Instead, endeavor to exchange, or if nothing else spread them with the goal that your days are relatively even.

- For example, if you are completing two days of high carbs and five days of low carbs, you may feel enticed to make both Saturday and Sunday high-carb days. Be that as it may, it would be better if you spread these two days out. For example, you could make Tuesday and Saturday your high-carb days.

4 *Think of a dinner plan.* One of the best ways to remain on track with your carb cycling is to the thought of a super strategy for every day. Make a nitty-gritty arrangement concerning what you will eat for every day of the week. Having a clear plan will help keep you on track.

An example of a low-carb day feast plan could resemble this:

- For breakfast, two fried eggs in addition to half of a ringer pepper.
- As a morning nibble, you can have a protein shake and a bunch of berries (for example raspberries, strawberries, blackberries, etc.)
- For lunch, have three ounces of barbecued chicken with one cup of asparagus.
- For an evening nibble, have 33% of a cup of oats (cooked) with ten almonds.
- Have a three-ounce steak with two cups of steamed broccoli or cauliflower for supper.

For a high-carb day, your dinner plan may resemble this:

- Half a cup of cereal with walnuts and berries of your decision for breakfast
- As an early in the day nibble, appreciate an apple with two tablespoons of nut butter (for example peanut butter or almond butter).
- Half of a turkey sandwich on whole grain bread for lunch.
- As an evening nibble, eat one cup of three beans serving of mixed greens with one cup of quinoa.
- For supper, attempt three ounces of flame-broiled chicken with one cup of whole wheat pasta beat with pesto.

5 *Screen your advancement.* It is essential to watch out for your improvement to perceive what is working and what isn't working so you can alter appropriately. If, after sticking to a schedule for a couple of weeks, you haven't seen any improvement, at that point, you may need to alter your carb cycling schedule. For example, if you've been eating low-carb for four days every week and high-carb for three days every week, you should need to have a go at changing to five days of low-carb and two days of high carbs.

- Additionally, take a gander at the things you are eating. This diet depends on having a healthy eating lifestyle and is certainly not a convenient solution all. On your high-carb days, you ought to eat good sources of carbs, for example, organic products, whole grains, and vegetables. On your low-carb days, you should at present be practicing good eating habits. Fish and lean meats, for example, chicken are a good source of protein, which will help shield you from inclination hungry. In addition to that, you can eat leafy green vegetables that are low in carbs.

Staying Healthy

1 Converse with your doctor. For certain people, eating a low-carb diet may be beneficial for managing other medical issues; in any case, there may likewise be some medical issues that could be exacerbated by a low-carb diet. Along these lines, it is a good idea to converse with your doctor about carb cycling before starting the diet.

- This is valid for any significant lifestyle change, not merely carb cycling. It is essential to figure out how specific lifestyle changes may interact with any wellbeing conditions you may have before taking them on.

2. Attempt to ensure your carbs are good carbs. Typically, carb cycling diets don't limit what you can and can't eat. Nonetheless, it makes sense that when you do eat carbs, you should go for sustenances that are solid and natural. For example, nourishment, for example, rice, potatoes, whole grain bread, vegetables, and other whole grains all give an excellent wellspring of sound carbs.

- These are otherwise called safe starches.
- A few people likewise prescribe restricting yourself specifically to what is called "complex carbohydrates." This is in contrast with refined carbohydrates, which are usually very handled and don't contain much fiber. Examples of complex carbohydrates incorporate whole grains, organic products, vegetables, beans, vegetables, and nuts. These will be handled by your body all the more slowly and will keep you feeling full for longer.

3 Allow yourself an occasional treat. To adhere to any diet over the long-term, you'll need to allow yourself a reward. If you don't, you will more than likely get baffled and surrender. Hence, you ought to allow yourself a cheat meal once every week. This doesn't mean an all-out binge meal, however if you need to have a dessert with your meal or something that you usually wouldn't eat, at that point allow yourself to have it.

- When you have your reward, attempt to relish it, don't only eat it all down without tasting it.

4 Try not to skip breakfast. If you are on a low-carb day, you may imagine that an easy way to remove some carbs (and calories) is to skip breakfast. Be that as it may, you ought not to skip breakfast regardless of whether it is a low-carb day or a high-carb day. Having breakfast is vital for your overall prosperity, and it regularly helps get thinner.

- If you don't possess much energy for breakfast, keep it basic. You can make oatmeal in a microwave in just a couple of minutes. If you are running late, grab a banana.

5 Perceive issues. The idea behind carb cycling is to anticipate the negative side effects that may occur because of a low carb diet. So, there are risks that accompanied not getting enough carbohydrates in your diet, and some negative side effects may occur. If you notice any of the following symptoms, you may need to change your carb cycling schedule to adjust your diet.

- Cerebral pains, shortcoming, terrible breath, feeling tired, and blockage or looseness of the bowels may all occur if your body isn't getting sufficient carbohydrates.

Understanding Carb Cycling

1. Know that carb cycling is intended to be more comfortable on the body. Carbohydrates have gotten a bad reputation in the last quite a long while. Lamentably, this bad reputation isn't generally merited because carbohydrates assume a huge role in keeping your body working and sound. Limiting your carbohydrates over the long term can affects affect your body. In this manner, utilizing carb cycling, you can give your body the carbs it needs to continue onward while as yet getting more fit.

Carbohydrates are a primary fuel for your body. Without this fuel, your body slows down so it can preserve energy.

For instance, long-term carb confinement can make the metabolism, in reality, slow down.

2. Comprehend that carb cycling can avoid levels. Regardless of whether your goal is to gain muscle, to lose fat or both, many fitness professionals trusts that carb cycling offers a decent method to shield your body from leveling. Consequently, if you feel that you are having an increasingly difficult time gaining muscle, or losing that last five pounds, a carb cycle may help get you over that level.

This is because while you are eating a low-carb diet, you are likewise "astonishing" your body with a couple of days of high-carb consumption. This keeps your metabolism from slowing down.

3 Comprehend that carb cycling likewise implies calorie cycling. When that you eat more carbs, you will likewise be eating more calories, and that is ok if your carbs are originating from sound sources. This is because carbohydrates usually are more calorie thick. When that you are eating low carb, you will generally consume fewer calories as long as you are sticking to sound nourishments (for example lean meat, fish, and loads of leafy greens).

This is particularly essential to comprehend if you are attempting to get in shape since you might be stressed that you are eating such a large number of calories on your high-carb days. In general, if you are sticking to solid high-carb meals with reasonable portion sizes, at that point, those additional calories won't be an issue.

Tips

Comprehend that eating healthy is important for shedding pounds, just as for generally speaking health. Be that as it may, you should keep up a regular exercise routine too whether your goal is to get more fit, or if it is to pick up muscle.

Get that while numerous individuals use carb cycling as a weight misfortune technique, most (however not all) explore on this strategy has been directed on rodents.

This technique may not be appropriate for everybody. If you have health conditions, you should converse with your doctor about carb cycling before rolling out any huge improvements to your dietary patterns.

Carb cycling diet plan

There aren't many controlled examinations straightforwardly exploring a carb cycling diet.

Carb cycling endeavors to coordinate the body's requirement for calories or glucose. For example, it gives carbohydrates around the exercise or on full training days.

The high-carb days are additionally set up to refuel muscle glycogen, which may improve execution and lessen muscle breakdown.

Vital high-carb periods may likewise improve the capacity of the weight-and hunger directing hormones leptin and ghrelin.

The low-carb days are accounted for to switch the body over to a dominatingly fat-based vitality framework, which may improve metabolic adaptability and the body's capacity to burn fat as fuel in the long-term.

Another huge component of carb cycling is the control of insulin.

The low-carb days and focusing on carbs around the exercise may improve insulin affectability, an essential marker of wellbeing.

In theory, this methodology will augment the advantages carbohydrates give.

Although the systems behind carb cycling bolster its utilization, it ought to be translated with alert because of the absence of direct research on the methodology.

Will Carb Cycling Help You Lose Weight?

The mechanisms behind carb cycling suggest that it very well may be gainful for weight misfortune.

In theory, carb cycling may enable you to keep up physical execution while giving a portion of the same advantages from a low-carb diet.

Similarly, as with any diet, the fundamental component behind weight misfortune is a calorie shortfall, as in eating not correctly, your body burns over a prolonged timeframe (16 Trusted Source).

If a carb cycling diet is executed alongside a calorie deficiency, at that point you will probably get in shape.

Notwithstanding, its increasingly perplexing nature may cause adherence issues and disarray for fledglings.

Conversely, numerous people may appreciate the adaptability of carb cycling. This could probably improve adherence and long-term accomplishment for certain people.

Carb Cycling for Muscle Growth and Sports Performance

Numerous people trust that carb cycling can be useful for muscle gain and physical execution.

The regular high-carb periods and focused on carb intake may help improve execution.

Carbs around the exercise may likewise help with recuperation, supplement conveyance, and glycogen recharging.

This may likewise advance muscle growth. In any case, some research suggests carbs are not expected to build muscle if protein intake is enough.

While these mechanisms bode well in theory, direct research contrasting carb cycling with different diets is expected to give a proof-based answer.

Does Carb Cycling Have Any Other Benefits?

As of now mentioned, carb cycling can give a few advantages that different diets can't.

By having times of low and high carb, you may get a significant number of the advantages given by the two diets, without a portion of the negatives.

Advantages of low-carb periods may incorporate better insulin affectability, expanded fat burning, improved cholesterol, and upgraded metabolic wellbeing.

High carb refeeds may likewise effects affect hormones amid a diet, including thyroid hormones, testosterone, and leptin.

These variables may assume an essential job in long-term dieting achievement since hormones believe a key role in yearning, digestion, and exercise execution.

Example Carb Cycling Menu

Here are three sample meal plans for low-, moderate-and high-carb days.

High-Carb Day

- Breakfast: 3 bubbled eggs, 3 cuts Ezekiel (or 7 seed/grain) bread, tomatoes, mushrooms and a side bowl of the blended organic product (60 g carbs).
- Lunch: 6 oz sweet potato, 6 oz lean meat or fish, blended vegetables (45 g carbs).
- Pre-Workout: 1 serving oatmeal, almond milk, 1 glass berries, 1 scoop whey protein (50 g carbs).
- Supper: 1 serving whole meal rice, 6 oz lean chicken, natively constructed tomato sauce, 1 serving kidney beans, blended vegetables (70 g carbs).

Moderate-Carb Day

- Breakfast: Grass-bolstered high-protein yogurt, 1 glass blended berries, stevia, 1 spoon seed blend (25 g carbs).
- Lunch: 6 oz chicken plate of mixed greens with 4 oz diced potatoes (25 g carbs).
- Pre-Workout: 1 banana with a whey protein shake (30 g carbs).
- Supper: 1 serving sweet potato fries, 6 oz lean meat, natively constructed tomato sauce, 1 serving kidney beans, blended vegetables (40 g carbs).

Low-Carb Day

- Breakfast: 3 eggs with 3 cups of bacon and blended vegetables (10 g carbs).
- Lunch: 6 oz salmon plate of mixed greens with 1 spoon olive oil (10 g carbs).
- Bite: 1 oz blended nuts with 1 serving turkey cuts (10 g carbs).
- Supper: 6 oz steak, half avocado, blended vegetables (16 g carbs).

Recommended Carbohydrate Food Sources

A few carbohydrates ought to be dodged, aside from on different events or for the seasonal treat.

Interestingly, there are a lot of healthy carb sources that are delectable and stuffed loaded with advantageous fiber, vitamins, and minerals.

When arranging your high-carb days, don't blame it for a hard and fast pop-tart gorge. Instead, center around these healthier carb choices.

Recommended "Good" Carbs:

- **Whole Grains:** Unmodified grains are fit as a fiddle and connected with numerous medical advantages. Sources include brown rice, oats, and quinoa.
- **Vegetables:** Every vegetable has a different vitamin and mineral substance, eat an assortment of hues to get the right balance.
- **Natural Fruits**: As with vegetables, every organic product is one of a kind, particularly berries with their high cancer prevention agent substance and low glycemic load.
- **Vegetables:** An incredible decision of slow processing carbohydrates, which are loaded with

fiber and minerals. Ensure you set them up appropriately.

- **_Tubers:_** Potatoes, sweet potatoes, and so on.

CHAPTER FOUR

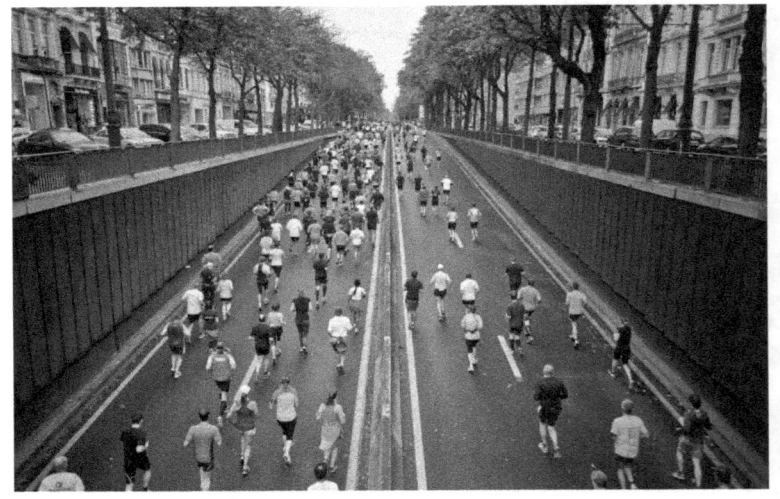

Carb Cycling For Weight Loss

Here's the ish with carbs: You need them to control through muscle-building workouts, however eating too many can add to fat stockpiling and overabundance pounds.

That is the reason a few specialists state that carb cycling for weight reduction or boosting your carb intake some days and decreasing others, maybe the happy medium we've all been searching for. Here, we dive into whether this popular way of eating can enable you to drop pounds without surrendering the best nutrition class.

What Carb Cycling Means

There are a ton of carb-cycling regimens out there. For example, some serious athletes, similar to bodybuilders, who know exactly when and to what extent they'll work out every day pursue a week after week design. That may incorporate a high-carb day pursued by three days of eating almost no carbohydrates. For these kinds of plans, dieters monitor every gram of carbs they expend,

The exact amount of carbohydrates they eat thoroughly relies upon their weight, muscle mass, objectives, and action levels, he says. Be that as it may, for the average active woman hoping to get more fit, the best way to take on carb cycling is on a day-to-day premise,

How It Works

On days when you're smashing it at the exercise center or preparing for a race, carbs are your BFF. Your body burns through them (alongside fat) for energy rather than protein. That permits the muscle-building nutrient to focus on carrying out its responsibility.

But, on days when you don't leave the lounge chair, eating extra carbs could urge your body to store that unused glucose in your fat cells. By eating fewer carbs on a rest day, your body turns to fat for energy rather than the sugary and dull sustenance it, as a rule, eats up.

Would it be able to Help You Lose Weight?

For those days when you're playing work area racer or habitually lazy person, there are unique weight reduction benefits to chowing on fewer carbs. "You don't should store all these extra calories if they're not going to be utilized," says Fear. "In contrast to your fat and protein admission, your carb needs vary starting with one day then onto the next." Also, when you swap carbs for protein and veggies, it ends up trickier to indulge (the more significant part of us don't gorge on broccoli and chicken), so helps your waistline.

Would it be a good idea for you to Try It?

While there's nothing hazardous about exchanging up the way you expend carbs, "estimating things down to the gram places you in a restrictive mindset, which can abandon you needing that sustenance you're passing up," says Fear.

Arb cycling without a lot of gram guidelines appears as though it would be less compelling (particularly contrasted with the plans bodybuilders pursue). In any case, since everyone's needs are different, sticking to one-size fits all strategy isn't the best technique for gathering your weight reduction objectives,

So, Fear outlines how to make a carb-cycling diet work for you.

What a High-Carb Day Resembles

On an average day, around 60 percent of your calories should originate from complex carbs. That is about 900 calories in case you're eating 1,500 calories per day.

On high-carb days, when you've planned a high-energy workout, as metabolic molding, interim preparing, runs, or a long-separate run, include an extra serving or two of whole grains, organic products, or vegetables. "In case you're gassed 10 minutes into your workout, you should take a stab at including another serving,".

What a Low-Carb Day Resembles

On days when you don't work out at all or accomplish something relaxed, such as running for 30 minutes or taking a hatha yoga class, have a go at swapping a serving or two of your regular carb consumptions with green veggies, lean protein, or solid fats. For example, if you usually have a whole-wheat turkey sandwich for lunch, attempt a turkey and spinach salad with cheddar.

The bottom line: It's essential to keep away from a transactional mindset about nourishment, says Fear. Musings like, "I ran an extra mile so I can eat this," are a slippery slope to an unfortunate association with sustenance.

All things considered, "having higher carbs on some days and lower carbs on different days are how the body normally controls itself," says Fear. "So, there's nothing wrong with exploiting a portion of the benefits of lessening carbs."

Your Carb-Cycling Meal Plan

Need out carb cycling for weight reduction an attempt? Pursue this week-long carb-cycling meal plan, politeness of Fear. On higher-carb days (Monday, Wednesday, Friday, Sunday), perform high-intensity or long-span workouts. Choices incorporate interim preparing, runs, lifting, or long runs. On lower-carb days (Tuesday, Thursday, Saturday), rest or perform lower-intensity workouts like yoga, barre, or light running. You should feel fulfilled, yet not stuffed, after every meal. If you aren't, increment your portion sizes or include a bite.

MONDAY: HIGHER-CARB DAY

Breakfast: 1/2 cup outdated oats cooked with 1 cup 1% milk, an apple or banana, and 2 tablespoons slashed walnuts. (443 cals, 67 g carbs, 16 g protein, 15 g fat)

Lunch: Sandwich with 2 slices whole-wheat bread, 4 ounces store turkey, 1/5 medium avocado, and mustard. 3 ounces raw carrots and 2 tablespoons hummus as a side. (385 cals, 53 g carbs, 26 g protein, 11 g fat)

Dinner: 2 ounces whole-wheat pasta hurled with tomato-basil sauce, cut zucchini, and 4 ounces lean ground hamburger. 1/2-ounce dark chocolate for pastry. (661 cals, 57 g carbs, 41 g protein, 32 g fat)

TOTAL: 1,489 cals, 177 g carbs, 83 g protein, 58 g fat

Optional snack: 2 whole grain crispbreads with 2 The Laughing Cow Swiss cheddar wedges (140 cals, 12 g carbs, 5 g protein, 8 g fat)

TUESDAY: LOWER-CARB DAY

Breakfast: 2 egg whites in addition to 2 eggs mixed with one bunch infant spinach and beat with one cut mozzarella cheddar. 1 cup strawberries as a side. (317 cals, 20 g carbs, 27 g of protein, 14 g fat)

Lunch: Spinach salad beat with 4 ounces cooked wild salmon, low-starch veggies (tomatoes, cucumber, peppers), 2 teaspoons olive oil, and 2 teaspoons balsamic vinegar. 6 ounces Greek yogurt (light or plain low-fat, without included sugars) as a side. (388 cals, 19 g carbs, 42 g protein, 7 g fat)

Dinner: 4 ounces flame-broiled chicken breast with 1/2 cups roasted asparagus and 1 cup butternut squash, cooked with 2 teaspoons olive oil. (323 calories, 24 g carbs, 33 g protein, 11 g fat)

TOTAL: 1,028 calories, 63 g carbs, 102 g protein, 32 g fat

Optional snack: 1 hard-bubbled egg. (71 cals, 0 g carbs, 6 g protein, 5 g fat)

WEDNESDAY: HIGHER-CARB DAY

Breakfast: Parfait of 6 ounces low or nonfat Greek yogurt, 1/4 cup granola, 1 chopped pear, 2 tablespoons raisins, and 1 tablespoon ground coconut drops. (338 cals, 57 g carbs, 20 g protein, 4 g fat)

Lunch: Large whole-wheat tortilla loaded up with 1/2 cup refried beans, 1-ounce ground cheese, and salsa, lettuce, onion, and tomatoes. 1 cup grapes as a side. (530 calories, 71 g carbs, 19 g protein, 19 g fat)

Dinner: 4-ounce flame-broiled pork chop with 1/2 cup applesauce, 3/4 cup cooked brown rice, and 1/2 cups steamed broccoli with lemon pepper and 1 teaspoon spread. Side: a large portion of banana spread with 1/2 tablespoon nutty spread. (578 calories, 70 g carbs, 44 g protein, 14 g fat)

TOTAL: 1,446 cals, 198 carbs, 83 g protein, 37 g fat

Optional snack: 2 slight rice cakes topped with 1-ounce avocado, fresh basil, and salt. (99 cals, 17 g carbs, 1 g protein, 4 g fat)

THURSDAY: LOWER-CARB DAY

Breakfast: 1 egg and 1 egg white mixed with 2 slices turkey bacon (chopped) and 1/2 cup ringer peppers and onions. As an afterthought: 1/2 cup cottage cheese with 1 tablespoon all-natural product jam. (325 calories, 19 g carbs, 31 g protein, 14 g fat)

Lunch: 2 cups vegetable soup with 2 cups side salad (spinach, 1 cup tomatoes, 3/4 cup cucumber, 5 Kalamata olives, 3/4-ounce disintegrated feta, and balsamic vinegar). (358 calories, 56 g carbs, 14 g protein, 10 g fat)

Dinner: 6 ounces baked cod with tomatoes and oregano, 1 cup roasted green beans with 2 teaspoon olive oil, and 1/2 sweet potato with 1 teaspoon margarine. (381 cals, 31 g carbs, 41 g protein, 14 g fat)

TOTAL: 1,064 cals, 106 g carbs, 86 g protein, 38 g fat

Optional snack: 6 ounces low-fat Greek yogurt. (100 cals, 17 g protein, 6 g carb, 1 g fat)

FRIDAY: HIGHER-CARB DAY

Breakfast: Whole-wheat English muffin with 2 tablespoons almond margarine and 1 cut banana (419 cals, 56 g carbs, 13 g protein, 19 g fat)

Lunch: 2 cups lentil soup with a side salad (2 cups greens, tomatoes, and peppers with 1 chopped apple, 1-ounce ground cheddar, and 2 tablespoons vinaigrette). (530 cals, 77 g carbs, 27 g protein, 14 g fat)

Dinner: 8-inch whole-wheat cheese pizza (attempt Amy's) with a side of carrots, celery, and 2 tablespoons hummus (479 calories, 58 g carbs, 19 g protein, 20 g fat)

TOTAL: 1,428 calories, 191 g carbs, 59 g protein, 53 g fat

Optional Snacks: 1-ounce raisins. (27 cals, 7 g carbs, 0 g protein, 0 g fat)

SATURDAY: LOWER-CARB DAY

Breakfast: Protein pancakes (custom made or 1/2 cup Kodiak Cakes control cakes blend) topped with 1/2 tablespoons almond margarine and 1/2 cup cut strawberries. (360 calories, 41 g carbs, 19 g protein, 15 g fat)

Lunch: 4-ounce turkey burger topped with 1/5 medium avocado and 1 cut Swiss cheese, enveloped with lettuce leaves. Side: an apple or banana. (457 calories, 29 g carbs, 39 g protein, 23 g fat)

Dinner: 4 ounces Cajun (chicken breast with Cajun flavors), 1/2 cup dark beans, and 1 cup sautéed peppers and onions with 2 teaspoons olive oil (396 calories, 27 g carbs, 41 g protein, 13 g fat)

TOTAL: 1,213 calories, 97 g carbs, 99 g protein, 51 g fat

Optional snack: 8 almonds. (56 cals, 2 g carbs, 2 g protein, 5 g fat)

SUNDAY: HIGHER-CARB DAY

Breakfast: Breakfast burrito with 1 fried egg, 1/2 cup dark beans, 2 tablespoons salsa, 1 cut pepper jack cheese, and fresh cilantro enveloped by a large whole-wheat tortilla. Side: 1 orange. (452 cals, 50 g carb, 23 g protein, 17 g fat)

Lunch: Baked potato topped with destroyed rotisserie chicken (4 ounces), 1 cup cooked broccoli, and 1/4 cup ground cheddar cheese. (482 cals, 42 g carbs, 47 g protein, 13 g fat)

Dinner: 1 cup cooked quinoa or brown rice, 2 cups blended veggies, and 4 ounces lean meat strips pan-seared in 1 teaspoon sesame oil. (674 cals, 66 g carbs, 40 g protein, 28 g fat)

TOTAL: 1,608 cals, 158 g carbs, 110 g protein, 58 g fat

Optional snack: 1 cup applesauce with cinnamon. (102 cals, 27 g carbs, 0 g protein, 0 g fat)

Carb Cycling Meal Plan

There are many carb cycling meals plans out there; however, not every one of them will have the foods that you like on them. Along these lines, possibly it's an excellent opportunity to make one of your own. Here I will demonstrate to you what types of foods, and why they ought to go into your meal plans.

The carb cycling meal plans are best done on a 6 meal a day plan, along these lines you will have enough sustenance to fuel you, and keep your metabolism up, which is essential in this diet.

There are 3 essential days in the carb cycling diet:

- High Carb Day
- Low Carb Day
- No Carb Day

On the high carb day, you will have 4 meals out of 6, which will contain the same number of carbs as you need. Make sure to blend it up with some lean proteins, for example,

- white chicken/turkey meat
- fish (canned)
- Protein shakes with at any rate 40 - 50g of protein in them. Keep in mind, and you will need to go 1g/1 lbs of body weight when you devour protein. This will help keep up your muscle definition.
- curds
- and egg whites.

Those are the best proteins you can expend amid your run of the carb cycling diet.

On the low carb day, you slice back on the carbs to just a constrained 3 meals with any carbs whatsoever. All others will have none, only lots of lean proteins, and veggies.

Your proteins are essential on this day, as they will be a significant part of your diet, so don't hold back out.

On the no carb day, you will have NO to LITTLE carb intake by any means. The more significant part of the carbs will originate from the veggies, or protein that you will eat for the day.

As should be apparent all through those 3 essential cycle days, you need to keep up your protein intake. This is the thing that nourishes your muscles, without it, you lose them, and your metabolism drops like a stone. Since keeping your metabolism up all through the diet is the way to making it work, then that would imply that eating your appropriate intake of protein is the way to the entire thing.

Without the best possible protein intake at 1g/1 lbs of body weight, the carb cycling meal plan will be invalid and void. Since without it, there is no metabolism, because there is no muscle to begin it up. So, while on the carb cycling diet, please keep up the required intake of protein, along these lines, you will stand an opportunity in achieving your objective of a pleasantly characterized body.

What amount would you be able to lose with Carb cycling

At the point when done right, carb cycling can deliver a quick weight loss. However, it should be done well. Jayson Hunter claims that you can lose up to 15 lbs in a single month. It is best not to define your goals that high to stay away from disillusionment. Regardless of whether you shed 10 pounds in a month, this is still a fantastic weight loss.

Is Carb Rotation Easy

This program requires a dedication on your part to work. However, it isn't that hard because you get the chance to eat the right amount of nourishment while you're on it so you shouldn't starve. This is a plan that has worked for many people previously; thus, you ought to have accomplishment with it.

Alcoholic Drinks That Are Low in Carbs

Cocktails, lager, and wine can be high in carbohydrates and sugar. In case you're endeavoring to diminish your carb intake, yet at the same time need to appreciate the occasional drink, there are low-carb liquor alternatives.

You can even have liquor on the keto diet, particularly once you've got a few hints and traps for lowering the carb counts of your preferred cocktails.

For whatever length of time that you're mindful of the best (and most noticeably terrible) liquor for low-carb diets, you'll have the option to make the most of your preferred drinks with some restraint without getting off track with your eating plan.

Shots and Highballs

Although they're sourced from grain, pure spirits, for example, rum, vodka, bourbon, gin, and tequila have no carbohydrates (after the refining procedure, all that is left is the liquor).

Spirits can be filled in as a single shot, with ice, or with a mixer. If you utilize a blender that is naturally calorie and without carb, similar to at present and shining water or club soda, you can make a sans carb drink.

Other well-known mixers do include calories and carbs. However, many brands of tonic water, ginger ale, cola, and lemon-lime soda (7Up or Sprite) come in diet versions.

In case you're making a drink that is heavier on the mixer than the liquor, for example, a highball, utilize low-carb mixers to keep away from included carbs.

Carb Count for Spirits

- Whiskey   0 grams
- Tequila   0 grams
- Brandy   0 grams
- Dry Martini   0 grams
- Ridiculous Mary   7 grams
- Margarita   8 grams
- Cosmopolitan   8 grams
- Gin and Tonic   16 grams
- White Russian   17 grams
- Rum and Coke   39 grams

Cocktails

The most direct without carb alternative beside straight shots are spirits combined with carbonated mixers. If you lean toward cocktails made with sweeter mixers like fruit juice, there are ways to make these drinks lower in carbs.

Low-Carb Mixers

Citrus mixers like lemon and lime juices, as a rule, don't contribute much sugar, as a solitary drink doesn't require much. The exception is orange juice. While orange juice doesn't have significantly more sugar per ounce (3 grams) than different citrus juices (2 grams), you commonly utilize more OJ to make a drink than, state, lemon or lime juice.

A standout amongst the most popular drinks made with OJ is a screwdriver (vodka and orange juice). Contingent upon the size, a screwdriver can without much of a stretch have 24 grams of carbs or more.

What You Can Eat on Phase 1 of the South Beach Diet

The carbs in other famous fruit juice mixers shift however remember that the amount you use (a sprinkle versus a pour) will impact your cocktails' last carb tally.

Carb Count for Fruit Juice Mixers

- Diet cranberry juice cocktail   0.2 grams
- Tomato juice   1 gram
- Light cranberry juice cocktail   1 gram
- Apple juice   3.5 grams
- Pineapple juice   4 grams
- Cranberry juice cocktail
- Artificial Sweeteners

Simple syrup is an answer of sugar in water used to sweeten cocktails. One ounce has 4 tablespoons of sugar, around 50 grams of carbohydrates and just about 200 calories. Simple syrup is regularly joined with lemon juice or lime juice to make a sweet-and-sour mixer.

To lighten the sugar and carb load, make your very own sans sugar sweet and sour mixer utilizing an artificial fluid sweetener. However, there are upsides and downsides to using artificial sweeteners you ought to consider before adding them to your alcohol bureau.

For instance, the principle intrigue of sugar substitutes is that they don't include calories or carbohydrates, settling on them mainstream decisions for individuals endeavoring to get in shape or control their glucose. Many products used to mix alcoholic beverages, similar to diet soda, powder mixes, and drops (like Crystal Light), have without sugar assortments.

However, to make up for the absence of flavor, artificial sweeteners are commonly a lot sweeter in taste than natural sugar. Some research has demonstrated that when we eat these more delicious sugar substitutes routinely, it might change our preferences. We may begin to like and search out sweeter foods, finding those with just naturally occurring amounts of sugar (or no sugar) excessively tasteless.

If you need to keep away from the added substances, search for products sweetened with stevia, erythritol, and fruit juice condensed or crystals.

Other Cocktail Ingredients

Small amounts of sharp flavoring, an alcoholic arrangement made with organic fixings, are regularly utilized in cocktails, unusually an Old Fashioned. Carb counts for great seasoning fluctuate. A few methods have few or no carbs, while different mixes can have upwards of 15 grams for each tablespoon.

Vermouth is a seasoned strengthened wine used to make exemplary martinis. Dry vermouth contains around 1 gram of carbs per ounce, while sweetened forms contain about 4 grams for each ounce.

Low-Carb Cocktail Recipes

- Low-Carb Cosmopolitan Recipe (1 gram)
- Sugar-Free Whiskey Sour Recipe (2 grams)
- Low-Carb Tom Collins Recipe (2 grams)
- Sugar-Free Margarita Recipe (6 grams)
- Tomato juice and vodka Recipe (9 grams)

Beer

Regular beer contains about 12 grams of carbs per serving. Notwithstanding, the number can vary, starting with one brand then onto the next, so check the name. In general, the darker or heavier the beer, the more carbs it has.

Craft Beer

The carb grams in 12 ounces of light beer varies from 2.4 to 7. Ales have around 5 to 9 carb grams. Stouts or dull beers differ significantly. However new stout varieties can have as much as 20 grams for each container. Check the mark or brewer's website for specific craft beers, however, remember that many can equal stout in carb tallies.

Beer Carb Counts

- Bud Select 55   1.8 grams
- Mill operator 64   2.4 grams
- Michelob Ultra   2.6 grams
- Mill operator Light   3.2 grams
- Coors Light   5 grams
- Bud Light   6.6 grams
- Heineken   11 grams
- Budweiser   11 grams
- Pabst Blue Ribbon   12 grams
- Stella Artois   13 grams
- Corona Extra   14 grams
- Guinness Extra   14 grams
- Fuller's London Porter   20 grams
- Samuel Adams Double Bock   27 grams

*by the container

Non-alcoholic Beer

If you like the flavor of beer however incline toward non-alcoholic adaptations, some are moderately low-carb and low-calorie. For example, a 12-ounce container of Busch NA Low Alcohol Beer has 60 calories and 12.9 grams of carbs, and MillerCoors non-alcoholic beer has 58 calories and 12.2 grams of carbs per 12-ounce can.

Wine

Generally speaking, wine contains a little measure of carbohydrate. While the carb means each type varies, as a general guideline, sweeter wines have higher carb tallies.

Wine Carb Counts

- Dry champagne 2.5 grams
- Sauvignon blanc 3 grams
- Pinot Grigio 3 grams
- Chardonnay 3.1 grams
- Pinot noir 3.4 grams
- Shiraz/Syrah 3.7 grams
- Cabernet Sauvignon 3.8 grams
- Zinfandel 4.2 grams
- Rosé 5 grams

- Riesling 5 grams
- Muscat 8 grams
- Great wines 12-14 grams
- Late gather wine 20 grams

*per 5-ounce serving

Wine or soul coolers can have 30 to 40 grams of carb per bottle. In case you're eating (and drinking) low-carb, maintain a strategic distance from "breeders" and "hard lemonade" as these beverages are principally sugar.

A Word from Very well

You can appreciate an occasional mixed drink, beer, or wine as a component of a low-carb way of life. In case you're slicing carbs to manage diabetes, know that alcohol can make your blood sugar levels whimsical. The road where alcohol affects blood sugar is additionally impacted by several specific factors, for example, the type and measure of alcohol you pick, just as whether you've had something to eat.

Keep in mind that diminishing a beverage's carb check won't reduce the impacts of alcohol, so always drink capably.